DIET Ssshhh...

IT IS ONLY A FOUR LETTER WORD

The HOW-TO-BOOK for creating your own
personal diet program and
TAKING CONTROL OF YOUR LIFE

Sheri S. Fasbinder

DIET

Ssshhh... IT IS ONLY A FOUR LETTER WORD

It is time to
take control of your life

Copyright © 2006 by Sheri S. Fasbinder

ISBN: 978-0-578-00409-9

THE BOOK

DEDICATION

To all the terrific people who have helped me, by work or by deed or just by being there through my life long struggle of taking control of my life—you know who you are, and this book couldn't have happened without you. A thank you to my readers because you have chosen to read my story and may it help you take control of your life and loose the weight you have always wanted to loose *and keep it off.*

INTRODUCTION

Just start with the facts here. I have a weight problem. This is what I always tell myself. My problem is I gain weight very easy from the calories I put in my body. Always have been this way, as far as I can remember. I was about eight years old when I starting adding those extra pounds. Everyone wondered why, "she doesn't eat candy and junk food" said my mother to the doctors. So, "WHY"?? Well, of course they ran some tests. The best they could come up with was, you guessed it, my Thyroid. Well, yes of course they put me on medication. Everyone just expected the medication to make me stop gaining weight and magically take off what I had gained. But guess what, that did not happen. I just managed to stay a little overweight the rest of my child hood. That is, just enough to get teased by some kids, but not too much weight, as I was very active and into playing sports. It was not until I was in my early teens, when I became interested in boys, that I decided it was time to start DIETING.

Well, here is another chapter in the art of diets, of course, you guessed again, "normal" diets were not enough, I had to cut back even more. Thus we have the starvation plan.

I am sure most of you have been there too. And for the few of us who are, I call, Diet Challenged, when we starve ourselves, our bodies say, "what no food," "we will have to just store what she gives us and keep it". Therefore, it takes longer to loose weight.

That was the story of my early years, and it came with fainting, loss of hair, hunger pangs, and you guessed it again, I was not as "skinny-as-a-rail." I carried that "athletic build", and always hoping when someone said those words, it was a compliment.

I spent my young adult hood struggling with weight gain. Trying to avoid starving myself, so I would not faint, I managed to attempt and succeed with many "fad diets". I even tried that liquid drink that came in a 32oz. bottle, it was an 80's thing, only to find that I was far from having enough nutrition, I had no energy to do anything, but I lost weight! Only to, you know, you have guessed right again, I gained the weight back.

Throughout all these years, up to my mid twenties I was a yo yo dieter. I call it now a Do Do Dieter.

I had my children in my late 20's, two of them, back to back, a year and a half apart. Who ever said, "Chasing around 2 young ones

can make you loose that baby fat"? Must have been someone who would have lost their added baby pounds without that running around. Back to the world of "fad diets" again, lost that weight in six months, that was "too quick weight loss". A year and a half, it was back on with a vengeance.

Well, I am never one to give up. I did let myself get a little depressed, I call it "Way Post Part um Blues". I went to my favorite doctor, the man who delivered my babies, I think he doubled as a counselor. He made me realize, this is who I am, this wonderful body, my temple. Just take care of it, and it will take care of you. Take control of what has come your way. You are not and never will be "Skinny-minnie". This is okay!!!

Here I was 32 years old, 60 pounds overweight, and finally realizing no "fad diet" was going to be the end all to be all, (magical diet), to cure it all.

I was very lucky to have bought a house from a real estate person who left in my basement two large boxes of note pads. With those note pads I devised my new way of life. Or should I say my creativity exploded. I designed my own diet, my lifestyle change, my diet for life. I wrote everything down that I consumed, every day. It was tough when you went out to eat, now there are a lot of

restaurants that cater to lower calorie, lower fat consumption. I did it, some days I ate less than other days, some days I ate more, some days oops, I didn't know how many calories that were in that, or I didn't want to know. But you know what, and I know you guessed it again, I lost weight.

It took me two years to take that weight off. I continued, every day, writing down what I consume. This has become a way of life. It is so easy to write everything down, and if I don't write it down,

I feel like I have missed something. Now my life has been the gaining and losing of five pounds instead of 60 pounds. A much healthier fluctuation. I find it a much happier way of life, not frustrated starving myself or depriving me of my much loved dark chocolate.

I work out every day. I can count on one hand each year, since I was 32 how many times I did not work out. My exercise includes walking, biking, lots of tennis, lifting weights, and my favorite machine, it is called an Elliptical Machine. Now that I am nearing my mid 50's I bought myself a bosu ball, it is a half ball with a flat base on one side, it is great for stepping with lots of cushion , my older joints need this. You would not believe how much exercise you can do while watching TV too.

I still have some of those note pads left, and my husband travels a lot so he brings me home pads of paper from the hotels, I will be writing down my calorie intake for years to come.

Lately I have been counting my grams of protein and sugars. This helps me with my energy level. I find 60 to 80 grams of protein a day gives me the energy to function properly. This is the only fun way to diet. Creativity is your key. Always remember diet is just a four letter word.

WHAT DOES "DIET" MEAN?

Just what does the word "diet" mean, anyway? Well, let's take a look at the dictionary:

diet \di-et\ (n) 1. a regimen of special or limited food and drink chosen for health or to lose or gain weight (vb) to eat or to cause to eat special or limited food, especially for losing weight.

This regimen that I'll be describing in this book is all about counting calories and losing weight at a slow, healthy pace. This, for me, has proved to be the only surefire way of shedding those unwelcome pounds and keeping them at bay. I don't think I'm being overconfident in predicting that it will work for you, too. I'll be offering plenty of tips and rules for healthy eating habits and a healthy lifestyle.

I'm not skinny, and I never will be--and that's okay with me. The best I can do is to keep myself about ten pounds above the "recommended" weight for someone my age and height. But the "average" person to whom that weight applies is not me, with my own build, my own medical history, my own metabolism. And chances are that is not you, either.

Who wants to be "average", anyway? Wouldn't you much rather be a healthy, happy, one-of-a-kind YOU?

My goal in writing this book is to make that you happen. As I guide you along the path I took, you will learn to understand your own body and what reasonably to expect of it. Every body gains and loses weight differently: every metabolism is unique. You've got to keep reminding yourself of that. Remember most of us were not meant to be "thin as a rail". But you also know most of us have tried to be this at some point in our life, and may still be looking to find that ultimate diet. The one that will make us lose all those unwanted pounds and keep them off. We have read the testimonials. We try it for ourselves, loose ten, twenty, and maybe
even fifty pounds--only to gain it back twice as fast as it took to lose it. We try it again, or we try another diet, only to lose and gain again. Some of us give up . We are all definitely frustrated!

There is no "magical" diet. In pursuing that impossible dream, we're losing sight of the definition of the word "diet": "a regimen of special or limited food and drink, chosen for health or to lose or gain weight".

That's right, limited—and limits mean, control. And control doesn't stop, ever, even when you are down to the weight you were aiming for.

CONTROL: THE CHALLENGE —AND THE FUN

You know what foods and beverages you love to eat and drink. Well, you don't have to give them up—go ahead and enjoy them, but in moderation. Know your portions—that's one of the prime keys to weight-maintenance success. Know just how many calories there are in a given portion of a specific food. Know the number of grams of fat, and which kind of fat it contains. We do need fat in our diets mostly the type we get from items such as nuts.

Paying this kind of close attention to your portions of food and drink can take a little work. But hey...isn't it worth the effort, to be able to enjoy the things you really like, and still lose weight? Down with those fad diets that are always telling you "No, don't touch!"

It's a pretty simple formula: control your portions, lose weight. Control your daily intake and take control of your life. You can do it—I did!!

So...are you ready to forget that four-letter work "diet," with all its negativity, and restore to "diet" a healthy, happy, positive spin? If you are, then let's go!!

Remember that YOU are in control of your body, not some remote magician or guru. You can control your own pace and progress. You don't have to starve yourself—you're meant to enjoy food and drinks, not to let them make you miserable. A few little treats aren't the end of the world. This book invites you to personalize a get-real way of life— and one that doesn't ignore that three-letter work "fun".

Your diet should revolve around your own personal lifestyle. A slower weight loss usually achieves better results in keeping the weight off. It may take time to learn how to enjoy a moderate, controlled food-and beverage intake, just as it will take time to lose the weight you want to lose. But I've got confidence in you: you can do this!!

Stay strong. Don't neglect giving yourself a few pats on the back. Learning to control your intake is an art, so think of yourself as an artist —the highly esteemed designer of your own diet.
So now, fellow designers—grab those sketchbooks and pencils! It's time to get down to work.

THE DIET DIARY

Your next step, you will need a book or just a little note pad. We will call it our "*DIET DIARY*". Something you can easily carry with you. In this book you will write down everything you consume. You will have to include the amount of calories and fat too. You will have the numbers in front of you, so just add them up, and you will see what you really eat and drink in a day. Remember, most foods and beverages have the fat and calorie count on their label. Easy, easy for you. Or just look in a fat/calorie book, that is somewhere in your house. You know you were tempted at some point and bought one.

Just a little work. And really, you can just purchase foods that have the labels on them – wow, so easy to get you started.

So let's begin to take control of our life. We will show them we can lose weight and keep it off.

It is so simple and fun. Just measure, write and enjoy. Soon you will see yourself achieve the ultimate goal, weight loss that will stay off.

Keep your *DIET DIARY* with you at all times. This way, even if you have one little old cookie or half a glass of soda, you can write that down too. After a few days of writing what you have consumed, you will see what you really put into your body. Most of us will have to keep our calorie count between 1200 and 1400 per day to lose weight.

Along with the lower calorie count, your total grams of fat should also be below 60. Keeping the fat grams lower usually means you are eating lower calorie foods too.

Like more fresh veggies and fruits. And you know what that means; you can eat a few more things. So have fun experimenting with your foods. You may also find that women need the lower calories and men can usually go higher. Oh well, that's the way it is.

And if you love fresh fruits and vegetables like I do, well you are off to a great start with lots of food for energy and low calories and fat for the quickest weight loss. We do need the right foods to give our bodies energy, so remember to add plenty of protein and fiber and not too much sugar as it is a false sense of energy.

You do not want to deprive yourself; you want to teach yourself what your body can handle before you gain weight. You will have to start measuring most of your foods, especially if you want to

consume the high calorie or high fat items (the bad stuff). You are working toward a goal of altering your eating habits, not depriving or starving yourself. Remember this process may be slower but it is more likely to work for a lifetime.

I find you do not miss the bad stuff too much. We have to be honest. You know we will always miss some of the bad stuff, so go ahead and indulge, just once in a while. Again, never deprive yourself. You do not want to feel as if you are on one of those fad diets.

Remember to have some fun figuring out which foods are best for you with optimal weight loss. You know how much fun it can be to experiment with food. Remember again that we all lose weight at a different pace and we have to adjust the amounts we consume. So try to have fun figuring this out and not too much fun as you do not want to gain weight, right?

The only thing you should gain by this is confidence: the confidence that you have the knowledge of how to control your eating habits. This knowledge will take you through your lifetime and give you the power to always be in control of your diet.

Write it down, you will see for yourself what you consume.
So enjoy creating for your self a lifetime of great eating habits. I did it and you can too!!!!

TIPS FOR OPTIMIZED SUCCESS IN LOSING POUNDS AND A HEALTHIER LIFE

- Avoid empty calories, the no nutritional value foods and drinks
- Drink 8-10 glasses of water a day. Water not only helps fill your stomach, it hydrates your body and helps flush it of toxins. And ladies: it is great for your skin (face).
- Drink or eat 3 calcium products. Yes, you know: milk, milk, milk. For those who can't have milk, they make a lot of lactose free products now, so check your local grocery store. Yogurt is wonderful, plus high in protein too. They also make wonderful tasting chocolate soy milk now, and they make it in a light formula for those a little more concerned with their calorie count.
- Enjoy your choices of soy products available at your grocery store. Not only a veggie but high in protein.
- Soy milk is not only a calcium product, but high in protein too.
- Most calcium products have protein too – double the benefits.
- Cheeses are great too for protein and calcium, but watch the fat contents.
- Eat 4-5 servings of fruits and vegetables per day. Aim for your highest in antioxidants. Examples: all the berries for your

fruits, and oranges too. Also look for veggies that help you stay young looking - green beans, edamame and chick peas. And remember that beans include chili beans and baked beans too. You can aim for cancer fighting veggies like broccoli, cauliflower, cabbage and even brussel sprouts.

- Eat 2-3 servings of fiber products per day. For example, whole wheat breads, fiber cereal, oatmeal, or nuts which of course provide protein and good fat too.

- Consume as little as possible of processed or canned foods as they are too high in sodium, which should be lowered for optimal health. If you must have canned foods, rinse them off thoroughly. Products like tuna are canned, but great to eat. Just get the water packed cans, and rinse well. And something new I discovered for those of us that do not have easy access to fresh grapefruit: there is canned grapefruit, but it is packed with sugar water. Rinse it off thoroughly, and you can avoid some of those sugar calories of the syrup in the can. Avoid high fructose corn syrup.

- Consume protein, but avoid trans fats. The leaner the better helps your body stay young. Watch out for high fat meats.

- Keep alcohol consumption low; as it may relax you so much that it might just slow down your metabolism, so weight loss may be slower. If you must drink, then try to stay with a lite beer, or preferably red wine for optimal antioxidants. White wine is okay too. If you must drink rum, do it with a diet cola, or have vodka with one of the many brands of lite juices. No mixes, because it will count as double the calories. Remember to avoid empty calories!

- Watch serving sizes of all foods and beverages for optimal benefits for calories, fats, protein and sugar
- Avoid eating after 8:00pm.
- Remember to learn and enjoy!
- Always eat as many fresh foods as possible
- Break up you meals, eat up to 6 times a day

SEROTONIN BOOSTERS

("They Make Me Feel Good"

Products)

These are products to <u>really</u> watch how much you <u>really</u> consume.
Enjoying in moderation can actually help you feel good.
One serving size of these food choices can be beneficial, pick one or
two of these per day for optimal benefit, have fun alternate!

- Potatoes
- Avocados
- Nuts (almonds, walnuts, pecans, pistachios, cashews, and
  peanuts, preferably enjoyed in this order for optimal results,
  because of the amounts of calories and fat in a serving, it is a
  good fat though).
- Wheat or Grain type breads with cinnamon and honey, double
  benefits, sweet enough for dessert and a whole grain
- Red wine (preferably), or white wine
- Dark chocolate (they make a70% cocoa product that is
  wonderful). Milk chocolate is good, just not as beneficial.

DINNING OUT OR ON VACATION

Well, you will not believe it, but it is possible to ENJOY going out to eat, while you are trying to lose weight. So believe it or not, you can do it, whether you just want a night out, or you are on vacation.

First, the most important thing is portions.

The second is that you can ask your server to ask the chef "what is in this meal?" Then you will know about how many calories you will be eating, so you can record it in your DIET DIARY.

Try to stay with items that are not fried, sautéed, creamy, loaded in cheese or butter, casserole types or a Hollandaise sauce. Unless you want to just add 20 grams of fat and 200 calories to your meal, ask yourself "Do I really want to do this creamy sauce?" Those numbers I just gave you are low, and probably would be right if you ate half of your meal. And there is another key: "EAT HALF OF YOUR MEAL", and enjoy a little treat. Many restaurants make mini desserts now, or you can always settle for the mint at the door.

Now you have to figure when you are on the road, you may need to stop at some fast food place. Your best bet there would be any non-fried chicken, without any sauce or mayo, keep the lettuce and tomato, and eliminate half the bun. Wonderful taste, with less fat and less calories. Most fast food places have a list of their fat and calorie count for their foods. So go to it, enjoy, and stay low on those numbers. Your main objective while dining out or on the go, is to stay low enough so you do not gain weight. Later, when you get home, you can cut back on those calories to make up for it.

There are a lot of better choices out there too, such as at breakfast: chose the scone with fruit juice or milk, or yogurt or cereal with milk, or oatmeal with fruit and milk. Or for lunch, skip the cheese; add salsa, barbecue sauce, or mustard to sandwiches or single patty burger. Try a baked potato instead of those fries, and sour cream instead of butter.

Now if you want to hit a Mexican restaurant, well guess what? The guacamole is better than the sour cream, it is the good fat. For the main course, just do chicken, no cheese, flour or whole wheat tortillas, and plenty of salsa, it is a veggie too, right?

As far as Chinese or Thai places, you can go with any protein and veggie and brown rice. Ask, "what is in the sauce".

You can have pizza too, just ask for light cheese. You would be very surprised , you do not notice flavor change. The only change is that you don't have cheese stringing down your chin! Now if you must have meat, do bacon or chicken (instead of fatty meats like pepperoni and sausage), then add some veggies.

There are other places well advertised with their fat and calorie count, which say "we have a non-fattening sandwich for you". You know who they are. So have fun while you are out there. Just concentrate on not gaining weight.

- Ask your server questions. Don't be shy. Maybe they have half-portion meals.
- Order an appetizer for your meal.
- And you know, you have heard it over and over – eat slowly. Stop eating when the hunger is gone. Take it home. You don't have to eat all your food.
- Look for grilled, steamed, baked, broiled, seared it its own juice, or poached.

You should be a success at dining out! I do it and you can too!!

BUSY LIFE – MEALS ON THE RUN

BREAKFAST

- Throw 2 tablespoons of peanut butter on 2 slices of wheat bread and a piece of fruit.
- Bran muffin and a glass of milk.
- Oatmeal with fruit cooks in the microwave in two minutes.

Just a few of the things you can throw together in one or two minutes, and be out the door with food of substance to give you energy for your morning, and curb your hunger until lunch.

LUNCH

- A can of tuna packed in water and rinsed, dump in a whole wheat pita. Add some lettuce or tomatoes, and a piece of fruit for desert.

- Mozzarella cheese sandwich on wheat bread, and some lettuce and tomato, with a piece of fruit for dessert.

- And of course, peanut butter and jelly on whole wheat bread, and a piece of fruit for dessert.

Just a few of the things that are good for losing weight that you can eat on the run.

DINNER

Well, dinner is another thing. You are not going to be able to prepare this in 1-2 minutes. Unless you have already prepared it and warm in up in the microwave. There are many options, with your main objective to eat dinner as early as possible, as close to 6:00pm as possible.

Some choices are: grilled chicken, fish, or low fat burgers (yes, there is a brand out there), or even a veggie burger if you so choose. Microwave a sweet or regular potato. Make a salad (but be careful on the dressing). Microwave some veggies. Do a stir-fry. Cut up those veggies in the morning – cook with meat or tofu later. Spray your pan with a canned spray, not oil or butter.

Almost anything you cook can be prepared in the morning. Your choices are endless with this in mind. You can count the fat and calories when you make the meal and divide into portions. For optimal weight loss, eat dinner as early as possible with no late night snacking. I did it and you can too!!

If you must have dessert, well again, believe it or not, you have many choices. You will always be counting fat grams and calories, so you know what you have left for the day, if any, if you want to lose weight.

I suggest: one small piece of dark chocolate, or they make fat free pudding, or sugar free gelatin. You can make a small box of chocolate cake, cut into serving sizes, preferably in half servings again for optimal weight loss benefits. Eat one serving at a time for minimal calories, and low fat. Any small box flavor can be made. Enjoy!!

HOLIDAYS AND SOCIAL EVENTS

- We know this is really tough.
- Your main goal is not to gain weight.
- You must choose between desserts or drinks, not both in one day.
- If it is a dessert, you can ask what it is made from (sneaky idea!), like you want to make it yourself. Now you will have a general idea how much fat and calories are in it. If you made it yourself it is easy to get a general idea too.
- Your best bet is to stay away from saucy or fried foods, and things with lots of high calorie ingredients.
- If you have a general idea of fat and calorie count, you will know about how much it will take before you start gaining weight.
- Thanksgiving you can eat early. Make it 6 oz of turkey and they do make low fat gravy too. Have a cup of acorn squash and some green beans too. You can even have ¼ cup cranberry sauce. Then for that stuffing, you can do low fat on that too by adding low sodium cans of chicken broth instead of butter for the moisture.

- Saute your onions and celery for your stuffing in pan spray. Keep your portion to a cup. Then for your treat, how about a slice of pumpkin pie. AND EXERCISE
- If you fail at all the above, oh well, hope it was not too many days. Just pick yourself up, and restart your healthier lifestyle.

MEAL PLANNING FOR BREAKFAST

You know what you love to eat and drink, so enjoy these, but measure portions of each item you consume. This is a little work to begin with, but knowing you don't have to change your life completely to lose weight is the reward for this effort. A minor altering of food intake and achieving a way to keep the weight off for life is the ultimate goal.

Here are some great examples of a good low calorie day. You may want to start with something similar to what you already have for breakfast. Measure milk and cereal for a smaller serving size, sorry, not that free-pour amount. For most of us, we are concerned about our calcium intake, so if you don't have milk with cereal, how about a yogurt, or a glass of chocolate soy milk, which will also help satisfy that sweet tooth. Two to three servings a day of dairy can not only fill your stomach, but give yourself much needed calcium and protein. I think we all know why we need calcium: strong bones and protein for energy. So why not have a calcium product to start the day.

Have one egg and two pieces of center-cut style of bacon, and one piece of toast with lite butter, instead of scrambled eggs with cheese and sausage. And if you must have the cheese, have it with one egg and no bacon. Try a lite brand of cheese or go with parmesan, mozzarella or feta, which allow you to have a portion without a high calorie and fat count

Be creative for your sweet tooth. On your cereal, add some berries, or just cut up an apple, then dip with a mixture of cinnamon and honey or brown sugar. Add a serving of nuts, preferably walnuts or almonds. An excellent source of fiber and protein and a nice sweet satisfying taste.

You can go back to Breakfast On The Run for some choices, or how about yogurt with fruit and a serving of granola cereal. These are great for a nutritionally balanced meal.

There are low calorie pancake mixes and syrups, or you can try a whole-wheat pancake mix, easy to make: mix 1 ½ cups skim milk, 2 cups whole wheat flour, 2 egg whites, and one teaspoon baking powder. Mix and cook in a pan with using pan spray.

For your oatmeal, add cranberries or raisins. And oatmeal you know how they say, it's good for your cholesterol. Then add some milk or add some cinnamon too. Some say cinnamon is good for a faster movement of your metabolism. Don't forget about the honey too.

For a light quick breakfast, you might have 2 tablespoons of peanut butter, regular or crunchy. Spread this on a banana or an apple. Great tasting high nutrition to start the day, and quick too.

Now if you keep your first meal of the day including coffee with or without cream and sugar, a glass of milk, and/or juice to 400-500 calories, you are on the right track for not only giving your body an energy boost, but starting your calorie intake in a low level for your ultimate weight loss. Optimal benefit is to split this into two breakfast meals and get protein in one of these meals.

If you stay with the suggestions, you will find these foods are also lower in fat, which will also help in a speedier weight reduction. For those of us that have the time or are willing to make the time, a mere twenty minutes of any type of exercise will also get your metabolism moving for another step in optimal weight reduction, a great way to start the day.

There are many variations on foods for breakfast for optimal weight reduction, so go ahead, experiment with all the foods you enjoy, but keep your calorie count between 400 and 500. For most of us, the lower the better, so pick and choose wisely. Enjoy your morning meal. Remember too, the fresher the food, the better. Eating processed food is not the best way to achieve our goals. With fresh food, you usually will be able to eat more food for less calories and grams of fat.

MEAL PLANNING FOR LUNCH

For your second meal of the day you might want to give yourself more calories to work with. An option to go for would be 400 calories for breakfast, 500 for lunch and 400 for dinner. Eating more for lunch means more time in your day to wear off your extra calories. Optimal benefit is to split this meal in two also, and enjoy more protein for your energy level. You are learning what it takes for you to lose weight and then maintain a good weight.

So at lunch have a grilled chicken sandwich from your favorite fast food place. Ask for tomato & lettuce, and no mayo. Trim off the extra bread. They do have a list for calories and fat grams that are in their product. You can save yourself 50-75 calories and 4-5 grams of fat by trimming the bread and skipping the mayo. Make sure you add a piece of fruit to this meal, maybe something sweet enough to satisfy that dessert craving.

If you want to splurge on that salad, throw on some bacon bits, just measure. Another option is a serving of regular salad dressing mixed with some red wine and vinegar if you have a larger salad to cover, then mix well. If you add just a little dressing then toss your salad, you'll be surprised how far a little bit can go.

When it comes to lunch meats, remember the fresher the better. How about good old fashioned peanut butter and jelly, you can add cinnamon and honey to this too. This might be the time of day to have that scoop of ice cream. There are a few 'lite' styles of ice cream that are truly good tasting. You can have half the amount if you go with the regular. You choose, you need to create a happy food lifestyle. Always remember the fresher the better, and that usually equates with being able to eat more and stay low on those calories.

Have fun going through your calorie book, or just look in the aisles at the grocery store. There are hundreds of food items that have their calorie count on them. Some may be even in the frozen food section for a full meal plan. Just add a fruit or veggie and some skimmed milk. So enjoy your lunch, you have created it.

MEAL PLANNING FOR DINNER

Here we are, at our last meal of the day. Hopefully, you can work it into your schedules to eat this meal as early as possible. They say not to eat past 8:00pm, but for most of us, that may be a little late. I say, by 6:00pm. Hey, somewhere in between, if that is the best you can do. For those of us that are maintaining our weight, well, there may be a little more flexibility for you on time. Give yourself some time to wear off those extra calories. You do not want to gain weight. Optimal benefit again split the meal in two when you can by eating say your vegies and your calcium or bread an hour before you eat the rest, and exercise.

Choose your meal wisely. There are so many choices, we are so lucky, all the food that has the nutritional labeling listed on their package, so easy. You can eat plenty of veggies and maybe a little bread too. Include your protein, as in every meal. Remember some calcium too along with that bite sized cookie for dessert.

There is something I really enjoy making. This tastes great and it is extremely nutritious and has a few variations in the style it can be made. I hope you enjoy this as much as I do.

Start with canned spray (rather than with butter) an onion and a green pepper or a zucchini and an onion, or all these vegies. Whichever style you like better. These veggies are full of vitamins and are filling too. Yum, I love cooked onion.

This is especially good when you add a little garlic (found in a jar in the veggies section of your grocery store), and maybe a couple of tablespoons of parmesan cheese. A lite style of cheese is the best way to go, but it does add calories and fat, so watch the amount. You can add enough cheese for the nutritional value of protein and calcium. Add a piece of chicken or fish for more protein for your day. There is a whole wheat brand of pasta out there and this has extra protein too.

The basic recipe has approximately, with chicken, only 250 calories and 8 grams of fat. A perfect meal to have some left overs for another day when you might be in a hurry.

 So again have fun creating your menus. You know you have been doing your best when you are enjoying the food you eat while making it have lower calories and fat grams. So enjoy my suggestions and or create your own.

MEAL PLANNING FOR DESSERT

Now we all know this is something we should all avoid. But if you absolutely must…

I have included (later in the book) several great tasting lower calorie and fat count dessert ideas. These are based on you having one serving. You could consider having half of a serving too. The less the better here. Then there is the mini (bite size) candy bars too, all for approximately 50 calories and 2 grams of fat.

You can add some berries to a yogurt or 'lite' whip cream for a great dessert. And if you feel the need for a little more protein, add a serving size of walnuts. We are very lucky these days when it comes to dessert

There are so many items that have the nutrition facts right on their labels. So again, indulge yourself, but lightly. You are learning to change your eating lifestyle.   Follow the guidelines, don't stop at dinner you will have a healthy, happy diet lifestyle.

ONE WEEK MEAL PLAN

This seven day meal plan is a good way to get yourself started on a fat and calorie counting way of life. You can mix your days up to give yourself choices just in case you need to stay on this. Some of us may feel the need to have a plan set up for us. So I sure hope this will benefit you. All these meals are designed to be low enough for most of us to lose weight on. They are also balanced for optimal nutrition. Plenty of fruits and veggies. Protein and calcium and fiber products too. So go for it, good luck and stay strong. Remember, you <u>can</u> do it. Whenever possible save an item or two for between those meals, so you will ultimately be eating 5 to 6 times a day, for your optimal benefit.

Day 1: Sunday

Breakfast	Calories	fat grams
8oz glass of skim milk	75	0
1 cup 'lite' yogurt	100	0
½ cup blueberries	50	0
1 small egg	50	6
2 slices center cut bacon	<u>75</u>	<u>6</u>
	350	12

Lunch	Calories	fat grams
8oz lite orange juice w/ calcium	50	0
1 sour dough roll	100	1
lettuce & tomato salad	50	0
w/ ½ tbsp lite dressing	75	4
and 1oz feta cheese	75	6
1 chocolate sandwich cookie	<u>80</u>	<u>2</u>
	400	13

Dinner	Calories	fat grams
8oz glass skim milk	100	0
1 cup green beans	50	0
5oz lean sirloin steak	250	10
½ baked potato	50	0
2 tbsp lite sour cream	<u>50</u>	<u>4</u>
	500	14

Total:	**1250**	**39**

Day 2: Monday

Breakfast	Calories	fat grams
8oz skim milk	75	0
1 cup bran cereal w/ raisins	175	2
1 apple	100	0
1 slice lite banana bread	100	2
	450	4

Lunch	Calories	fat grams
Sandwich		
2 slices lite high fiber bread	75	2
1 slice cheese	100	10
lettuce & tomato, pickle	25	0
mustard	0	0
2 oranges	100	0
8oz skim milk	75	0
	375	12

Dinner	Calories	fat grams
8oz skim milk	75	0
½ baked chicken breast		
w/ BBQ sauce	150	6
2 cups cauliflower carrot medley	100	0
1 lite biscuit	100	2
	425	8

Total:	1250	24

Day 3: Tuesday

Breakfast	Calories	fat grams
1 serving oatmeal	150	2
8oz skim milk	75	0
½ cup blueberries	50	0
	275	2

Lunch	Calories	fat grams
2 slices high fiber lite bread	75	2
2 slices center cut bacon	75	6
lettuce & tomato	25	0
8oz skim milk	75	0
1 slice lite banana bread	100	2
	350	10

Dinner	Calories	fat grams
2 center cut pork chops		
w/ BBQ sauce, no fat, no bone	450	20
2 cups green beans	100	0
8oz skim milk	75	0
	625	20

Total:	1250	32

Day 4: Wednesday

Breakfast	Calories	fat grams
1 serving oatmeal	150	2
8 oz. Skim milk	75	0
½ cup blueberries		
with lite yogurt	125	0
	350	2

Lunch	Calories	fat grams
Salad w/ lettuce, tomato,		
Cucumbers, peppers,		
¼ cup cranberries, 8 walnuts	275	0
w/ 2tbsp lite dressing	75	4
2 slices lite banana bread	200	4
	550	8

Dinner	Calories	fat grams
½ chicken breast baked		
w/ BBQ sauce	150	3
2 cups broccoli, carrot,		
cauliflower medley	100	0
8oz skim milk	75	0
1 chocolate sandwich cookie	75	2
	400	5

Total:	1300	25

Day 5: Thursday

Breakfast	Calories	fat grams
1 small banana	100	0
1 tbsp peanut butter	100	9
1 'lite' yogurt	75	0
1 orange	50	0
	325	9

Lunch	Calories	fat grams
1 6oz can water packed tuna	150	2
Add peppers, onions, relish, and tomato	25	0
1 serving potato chips	125	10
1 chocolate sandwich cookie	75	2
8oz skim milk	75	0
	450	14

Dinner	Calories	fat grams
2 'lite' hotdogs	200	14
2 'lite' hotdog buns	150	2
1 serving baked beans	100	1
8oz skim milk	75	0
	525	17
Total:	1300	40

Day 6: Friday

Breakfast	Calories	fat grams
1 serving oatmeal	150	2
8oz skim milk	75	0
¼ cup raisins	125	0
	350	2

Lunch	Calories	fat grams
1 4"x4" piece of pizza w/		
pizza sauce, mozzarella cheese		
pepperoni and onions	275	12
1 apple	100	0
	375	12

Dinner	Calories	fat grams
Large salad – lettuce, tomato,		
Cucumber, peppers,		
1 serving mozzarella cheese	200	10
4tbsp dressing	150	8
½ cup blueberries w/ 2 tbsp		
of 'lite' whipped topping	100	2
8oz skim milk	75	0
	525	20

Total:	1250	34

Day 7: Saturday

Breakfast	Calories	fat grams
Pancakes (lite recipe, 1 serving)	225	5
¼ cup syrup	100	0
8oz skim milk	75	0
½ cup blueberries	50	0
	450	5

Lunch	Calories	fat grams
Sandwich – 2pc center cut bacon	75	6
Lettuce & tomato	25	0
2 slices high fiber bread	75	2
½ cup raspberries		
w/ 'lite' whipped topping	100	2
8oz skim milk	75	0
	350	10

Dinner	Calories	fat grams
8oz orange juice w/ club soda	100	0
6oz fish broiled (flounder, perch		
grouper or orange roughy)	200	6
½ baked potato w/		
1 tbsp sour cream	75	2
1 cup green beans	50	0
	425	8

Total:	1225	23

RECIPES

LITE BISCUITS

Preheat oven to 450°

1 ½ cups 'lite' baking mix

½ cup skim milk

Knead for 5 minutes

Spoon drop on can-sprayed cooking sheet

Bake 7-9 minutes at 450°

1 biscuit is about 100 calories and 2 grams of fat.

LITE PANCAKES 3-4" SIZE

2 cups 'lite' baking mix

1 egg

1 ¼ cup skim milk

Follow directions on box

225 calories and 5 grams of fat

Enjoy!

CREAMY TORTELLINI SALAD

Cook 9oz package of tortellini

Add 10oz package of snap peas to the last 2 minutes of boiling tortellini

In a separate bowl mix:

1 tbsp balsamic vinegar

1 tbsp 'lite' mayonnaise

1 tbsp grated parmesan cheese

12 cherry tomatoes

2 tbsp finely chopped onions

1 tbsp capers (optional), rinsed and drained

Combine with tortellini

Sprinkle with 2 tbsp of parmesan cheese

Serve warm or chill, then serve cold

1 ½ cup serving is approximately 200 calories and 8 grams of fat.

Enjoy!

PORK & CABBAGE SOUP

Sautee 1 tbsp olive oil with 1 garlic clove

Add 1 lb. pork tenderloin cut into 1 inch chuncks

Sprinkle with 1 tbsp sage

Sautee until cooked, then add 1 16oz package of coleslaw

Cook until coleslaw is soft

Add 16oz frozen mixed vegetables for stew

Add 4 cups low sodium chicken broth

Bring to a boil, reduce heat, cover for 10 minutes, stir occasionally.

Ready to eat. This is approximately 200 calories and 6 grams of fat for a 1 ½ cup size serving.

Enjoy!

BAKED RAVIOLI CASSEROLE

Preheat over to 400°

Spray 1 quart baking dish w/ can spray

Boil 9oz package of reduced fat cheese ravioli

and 2 cups cauliflower for 2 minutes

Drain and set aside.

Sautee 2 garlic cloves in 2 tsp olive oil for one

minute

Add 1 28oz can of diced tomatoes

Add ½ tsp Italian seasoning

Simmer for 5 minutes

Add ravioli mix and toss

Transfer to baking dish

Bake 20 minutes

This is about 250 calories for 1 cup and 2 grams
of fat.

Enjoy!

CHEESE BREAD

24 slices of French bread

Spread on each slice a mixture of:

2oz of softened Neufchatel cheese

½ cup 'lite' cheddar cheese

2oz jar of pimento

2 tbsp finely chopped pecans

½ tsp hot pepper sauce

Broil 4 in from heat 1-2 minutes

Each slice is approximately 85 calories and 2 grams of fat.

Enjoy!

STUFFED SHELLS

Cook 18 jumbo pasta shells

Stuff with mixture of:

10oz package frozen chopped spinach (thaw and drain)

8oz can water chestnuts (drain and chop)

¾ cup non-fat ricotta cheese

½ cup 'lite' mayonnaise

½ cup finely chopped carrot

3 tbsp finely chopped onion

¾ tsp garlic powder

¾ tsp hot pepper sauce

Each shell will use approximately 3 tbsp of the mixture

Refrigerate 12 hours before serving.

Each shell is approximately 150 calories and 4 grams of fat.

Enjoy!

LITE SAUCES

CARBONARA

2 4oz cartons egg substitute

2oz 'lite' Swiss cheese, shredded

1oz grated parmesan cheese

2 tbsp finely chopped chives

1 tbsp finely chopped Italian parsley

1 medium shallot, chop fine

2oz thin sliced 'lite' ham, cut into small pieces

Dash of pepper

Sautee ham in pan spray, then add other ingredients

Cook until sauce thickens – enjoy!

Makes 4 servings. Each serving is approximately 130 calories and 1 gram of fat each.

Enjoy!

ALFREDO

1 cup non-fat evaporated milk

¼ pound grated parmesan cheese

Pepper

Cook milk until it is at a simmer

Add pepper and parmesan cheese

Cook until thick and creamy

Divide into 4 equal parts

Each serving has approximately 150 calories and 7 grams of fat.

Enjoy!

CHILI CON QUESO

2 tbsp cilantro, finely chopped

1 tbsp peanut or corn oil

1 medium garlic clove, chopped fine

½ small jalapeno pepper, chopped fine

1 cup non-fat evaporated milk

6oz 'lite' cheddar cheese, shredded

4oz 'lite' Monterey jack cheese, shredded

Cook all ingredients except cheeses until creamy

Simmer 7-10 minutes, then gradually add cheeses

Stir until melted

Pour into 4 equal servings

Each serving has approximately 200 calories and 9 grams of fat.

Enjoy!

CAJUN SHRIMP JAMBALAYA

In a large skillet:

Heat 2 tbsp olive oil

Sautee 4 medium garlic cloves, chopped fine

1 small onion, chopped fine

1 green pepper cut into ½ inch pieces

Sautee for 5-7 minutes

Add:

1 pound small peeled & deveined shrimp

1 16oz can low sodium chopped tomatoes

1 tbsp tomato paste

2 tsp sugar

2 tsp oregano

½ tsp red pepper (cayenne)

¾ tsp ground cumin

1 bay leaf

½ tsp white pepper

½ cup Italian parsley

Cook until it thickens

Makes 4 servings with approximately 225 calories and 9 grams of fat. (Tastes great the next day, the way spaghetti sauce does). Enjoy!

SPICY EGGPLANT AND TOMATOES

Sautee in pan spray:

2 medium garlic cloves

½ tsp crushed red pepper flakes

½ tbsp basil

½ tbsp oregano

1 bay leaf

1 long thin eggplant, cut into small pieces

Sautee until bronzed

Add one 16oz can low sodium diced tomatoes

Cook until eggplant is tender and sauce has thickened (approximately 20 minutes). Enjoy!

Makes 4 equal servings, with 125 calories and 4 grams of fat each.

Enjoy!

MUSHROOM BARLEY SOUP

1 oz. dried mushrooms

3cups water

1 large onion chopped

2 carrots chopped

1 celery stick chopped

12 oz. can of button mushrooms

1 ½ tsp. oregano

2 cans fat free sow sodium chix broth

½ tsp. salt

½ cup barley

cook togerther 1-2 hours makes 6 sevings 150 calories, 1 gram of fat

Enjoy!

STUFFED MUSHROOMS

16 large mushrooms

1 small onion chopped finely

2 oz. Finely chopped spinach

2 garlic cloves finely chopped

1 can artichoke hearts finely chopped

½ cup parmesean cheese

3 Tlb. Lite mayonnaise

½ cup seasoned bread crumbs

¼ tsp. Red pepper

Bake 30 minutes at 400 degrees

8 servings 100 calories and 4 grams of fat

Enjoy!

APPLE CRISP

Preheat oven to 350°

6 apples, peel and slice

Sprinkle with:

    1 cup oatmeal

    ½ cup brown sugar

    ½ stick 'lite' butter

Bake at 350° for 45 minutes

This is a great low calorie, high fiber dessert with minimal sweet calories. A 6oz serving is approximately 150 calories and 4 grams of fat.

Enjoy!

BLUEBBERRY CAKE

Preheat oven to 350°

¾ to 1 cup sugar (less is good)

1 ½ cups reduced fat baking mix

1 egg white

1 whole egg

Mix

Spray bread loaf size pan with canned spray

Pour in mixture

Pour 1-1½ cups blueberries on top

Bake at 350° for 45 minutes

A 1" x 3" slice is approximately 75 calories, and 1 gram of fat.

Enjoy!

LITE BANANA BREAD

Preheat oven to 350°

1 cup sugar (1/4 cup for less calories with no taste difference)

1 ½ cups reduced fat baking mix

1 egg white

1 whole egg

2 large ripe bananas – mash

½ cup chopped nuts (optional)

Mix together

Spray 11" x 7" pan with canned spray

Bake at 350° for 45 minutes

A 1" x 3" slice is approximately 100 calories and 3 grams of fat. Without the nuts, it is approximately 80 calories and 1 gram of fat.

Enjoy!

S'MORE GORP

Preheat oven to 275°

In a large bowl mix:

2 cups honey graham cereal

2 cups low fat granola cereal

2 cups bran cereal squares

In a sauce pan melt:

2 tbsp 'lite' margarine

1 tbsp honey

½ tsp cinnamon

Pour over mixture in bowl, stir well

Spread mix on a large cookie sheet with sides

Bake 35-40 minutes

Cool completely, then add:

¾ cup mini marshmallows

½ cup raisins

¼ cup mini chocolate chips

Toss

½ cup is approximately 135 calories and 3 grams of fat.

Enjoy!

CRANBERRY MUFFINS

¾ cup all-purpose flour

½ cup whole-wheat flour

¼ cup yellow cornmeal

1 Tbl. Baking powder

½ tsp. Salt

½ cup plain fat free yogurt

½ cup fat free pasteurized egg substitute

¼ cup sugar

¼ cup maple syrup

¼ cup canola oit

2 tsp. Vanilla extract

1 ½ cups whole cranberries

Mix all together bake in sprayed muffin tin about 20 minutes at 400 degrees makes 12 muffins 150 calories 5 grams of fat

Enjoy!

Super Snacks – 100 Calories or Less

- ½ ounce fudge with or without nuts
- One tablespoon of peanut butter and 4 celery sticks
- One apple
- One cup of blueberries with lite whipped topping
- One cup chicken noodle soup
- 6 ounces of orange juice with 6 ounces club soda
- 24 pistachio nuts
- 7 animal crackers
- One peach
- One banana

- ½ cup of gelatin
- ½ cup lettuce with 2 tablespoons of salsa on a lite flour tortilla
- One cup of coleslaw with red wine vinegar and 1 teaspoon of sugar
- One ounce of pretzels
- One cup of microwave popcorn with butter
- ¼ pound boiled shrimp with 2 tablespoons cocktail sauce

Super Snacks – 100 Calories or Less

- 3 raw carrots
- ½ cup cooked eggplant with ¼ cup mozzarella cheese
- Alfalfa sprouts with 2 tablespoons soy sauce and 2 ounces of chicken
- One cucumber with red wine vinegar and 1 teaspoon sugar
- One lite yogurt
- One lite fruit smoothie
- One ounce cheddar or lite cheese
- One graham cracker
- One ounce of jelly beans
- ½ ounce of a plain dark chocolate bar
- One plain biscuit or crescent roll

EXERCISE

Now that you know what type of foods and beverages are good for your body type, you may want to find some exercise to do that will increase your chance for faster weight loss. You may want to contact your doctor first if you have never exercised or have any physical condition that would limit your activity. Exercise, for some this is a bad word, they just do not like it. For others it is the other key to weight loss success. For some it is a great way of relieving stress. Others find playing a sport, such as tennis or softball, or even bowling, is a great way to get exercise and relieve stress. Whatever your exercise will be, do it. You can purchase a video, such as yoga, great for tone and strength.

Find some through your doctor or local exercise facility to increase your chance for weight loss and weight maintenance. It is fun. I have heard many excuses over the years for not exercising, but boredom would have to be the number one funniest. My best suggestion for this is to exercise in increments of 20-30 minutes. Just 20-30 minutes of some type of exercise will help lead you down the weight loss path. Get started by putting yourself in the exercise mode by changing into exercise clothes.

Grab a book or thumb through a magazine, it is that easy. You will be surprised to see how fast 20-30 minutes goes by and in the long run you will be much happier with speedier weight loss results. Do check with your doctor on how much your heart rate should be elevated for your optimal health. For those of you that have no time for an excuse, well, the twenty minute thing can work for you. You will find how easy it will be as each day goes by to find twenty minutes to exercise. Before you know it you will be exercising once, twice, or maybe three times a day.

As far as this exercise thing goes, we all know how good it is for you. But did you know a brisk thirty minutes walk, 5-7 days a week may increase your life expectancy by six years, and reduce the risk of depression? Exercise, preferably with your heart rate elevated, is your best bet for optimal weight loss and overall body health. 30-60 minutes a day is optimal. Take your favorite pet for a walk too. Listen to some music, you will find yourself stepping to your music.

There are many of us that feel that we have to sit and watch the television after a long hard day at work. We have dinner, then sit. Well, as a little hint, how about some weights to curl while you watch TV? Or they have stretching bands you can purchase in your local department store's sports section. Or buy a simple machine that is made up with just a couple of pedals, so you can pedal like you're on a bike while you sit in your favorite chair. Even when you read the paper, you can stand and do leg lifts & curls with your weights.

Wow, are those simple ideas for exercise. All while watching TV. Before you know it, you will have exercised thirty to sixty minutes, without getting bored, even if "you don't have time".

They make portable stationary bicycles and treadmills. These are great forms of exercise, and you can read a book or watch TV while working out. Walk outside too, and grab a partner. You can have a great conversation with a family member or a friend and time zips right by. Talking is good for your lungs too. Weather permitting, grab your bicycle and pedal around the neighborhood for a half hour.

Remember, when you are sitting watching TV, grab some weights or those stretching bands. This will be good exercise for firming and loose skin by giving you muscle tone as you are losing weight.

This is also good for your bones, when you tone your muscles around them.

Well, you know how successful you can be with controlling your food and beverage consumption. Now you can show them how successful you can be at exercise!

CONCLUSION

- You are saying "Yes!" to everything in this book.

- Yes, weight loss is on my to-do list for the day.

- Yes, I am counting my fat grams and my calories

- Yes, I have a plan.

- Yes, I <u>will</u> stick to it.

- Yes, if I go off my plan, I will start again.

- Yes, I am committed to taking control of my life.

- Yes, I have found some exercise I like.

- Yes, I will stay active.

- Yes, when I reach my goal weight, I will stay at my goal weight.

- Yes, if I gain weight I will notice right away, and go back to my plan.

- Yes, I will not let myself get out of control again.

- Yes, I am in control of my life!

- Yes, I am an artist

- Yes, I will enjoy my new "Diet" life.

- Yes, I will treasure my DIET DIARY.

DIET DIARY

Date: _____

Food & Drink	Calories	Fat grams
Total		

DIET DIARY

Date: _____

Food & Drink	Calories	Fat grams
Total		

DIET DIARY

Date: _____

Food & Drink	Calories	Fat grams
Total		

DIET DIARY

Date: _____

Food & Drink	Calories	Fat grams
Total		

DIET DIARY

Date: _____

Food & Drink	Calories	Fat grams
Total		

DIET DIARY

Date: _____

Food & Drink	Calories	Fat grams
Total		

DIET DIARY

Date: _____

Food & Drink	Calories	Fat grams
Total